Jonas Salk and the Polio Vaccine

John Bankston

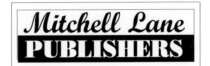

PO Box 619
Bear, Delaware 19701

Unlocking the Secrets of Science

Profiling 20th Century Achievers in Science, Medicine, and Technology

Jonas Salk and the Polio Vaccine

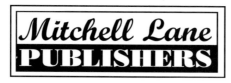

Copyright © 2002 by Mitchell Lane Publishers, Inc. All rights reserved. No part of this book may be reproduced without written permission from the publisher. Printed and bound in the United States of America.

First Printing

Library of Congress Cataloging-in-Publication Data
Bankston, John, 1974-
    Jonas Salk and the polio vaccine/John Bankston.
        p. cm. — (Unlocking the secrets of science)
    Includes bibliographical references and index.
    Summary: A biography of the scientist and humanitarian who discovered the vaccine for polio, a disease which crippled many people in the early part of the twentieth century.
    ISBN 1-58415-093-9
    1. Salk, Jonas, 1914—Juvenile literature. 2. Virologists—United States—Biography—Juvenile literature. 3. Poliomyelitis vaccine—Juvenile literature. [1. Salk, Jonas, 1914- 2. Scientists. 3. Poliomyelitis vaccine.] I. Title. II. Series.
QR31.S25.B365 2001
610'.92—dc21
    [B]   2001038096

ABOUT THE AUTHOR: Born in Boston, Massachussetts, John Bankston began publishing articles in newspapers and magazines while still a teenager. Since then, he has written over two hundred articles, and contributed chapters to books such as *Crimes of Passion*, and *Death Row 2000*, which have been sold in bookstores around the world. He currently lives in Los Angeles, California, pursuing a career in the entertainment industry. He has worked as a writer for the movie *Dot-Com*, which began filming in winter 2000, and is finishing his first young adult novel. In addition to being a writer, John is also a model and actor.

PHOTO CREDITS: Cover: Globe Photos; p. 8 Globe Photos; p. 10 Superstock; p. 16 AP Photos; pp. 22, 34 Archive Photos; p. 36 Globe Photos; p. 42 Archive Photos

PUBLISHER'S NOTE: In selecting those persons to be profiled in this series, we first attempted to identify the most notable accomplishments of the 20th century in science, medicine, and technology. When we were done, we noted a serious deficiency in the inclusion of women. For the greater part of the 20th century science, medicine, and technology were male-dominated fields. In many cases, the contributions of women went unrecognized. Women have tried for years to be included in these areas, and in many cases, women worked side by side with men who took credit for their ideas and discoveries. Even as we move forward into the 21st century, we find women still sadly underrepresented. It is not an oversight, therefore, that we profiled mostly male achievers. Information simply does not exist to include a fair selection of women.

Contents

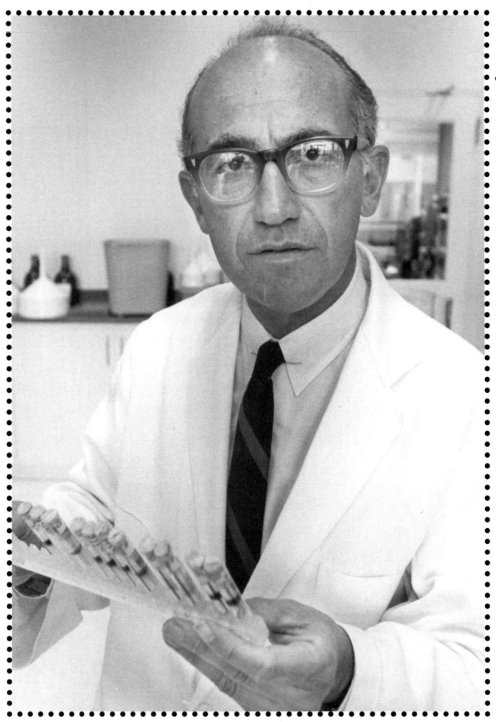

Going against popular medical opinion, Dr. Jonas Edward Salk developed the polio vaccine.

Chapter 1
Consequences

• •

The twentieth century was an amazing time filled with new inventions. From airplanes to computer chips, there was hardly ever a period in human history when so many discoveries altered the way that people lived. Yet even progress has a price.

Despite the advantages of these discoveries, there may also be drawbacks. These drawbacks are sometimes called "unintended consequences." For example, cars have improved travel, making it possible for people to go distances in a single day that used to take weeks. But cars also cause air pollution, which damages the environment. This is an unintended consequence.

In the late 1800s, as indoor plumbing and improved sanitation became more common, there was one tragic unintended consequence: polio.

Polio victims usually suffer permanent paralysis in their legs. Sometimes polio damages the muscles in the chest, and sufferers are unable to breathe on their own.

Polio is a disease caused by a tiny parasitic organism known as a virus. Viruses are so small they can only be seen with a very powerful microscope. The polio virus enters the victim through the mouth or nose, and settles for a time in the intestines before attacking either the spinal cord or the brain.

The disease is not a new one. The Greek physician Hippocrates described it over 2,500 years ago. Archaeologists have unearthed skeletons from nearly six thousand years ago which show twisted or bent leg bones, one sign of the disease.

Throughout history, despite occasional outbreaks, polio didn't claim very many victims. The illness was almost unheard of in poorer countries. It didn't become widespread until the end of the nineteen century and the beginning of the twentieth century in more developed countries such as the United States, Sweden, Great Britain, Norway, Switzerland and Canada.

In 1887, 44 cases were reported in Sweden. In Vermont's Otter Creek Valley seven years later, 132 children got the disease. Eighteen died. By 1905 there were more than a thousand cases in Sweden and several hundred in the United States.

Soon it was infecting even more citizens of these countries. It would take years of studies and claim tens of thousands of victims before scientists were able to learn why.

The explanation involves what are known as antibodies, which are cells that the body develops to protect itself from disease. Antibodies are formed for specific diseases. For example, a child may get chicken pox, which leads to the development of chicken pox antibodies. After the child recovers, he or she is forever protected—or immune—from a recurrence of chicken pox because of those antibodies.

The reasons for the increase in polio cases were directly related to hygiene and modern indoor plumbing. For most of history, when nearly everyone lived in very unsanitary conditions, babies were commonly exposed to the poliovirus before they were six months old. At that time in their lives, the disease would cause few—if any—

problems and they would almost always recover. As they recovered, they would develop antibodies and then have lifelong immunity from polio.

In the twentieth century that changed. By the early 1900s, many viruses like polio were reduced by indoor plumbing and an emphasis on hygiene or cleanliness. Babies no longer came in contact with the poliovirus on a regular basis, and never developed polio antibodies as infants. Consequently, when they were exposed to the polio virus later in life as older children or even as adults, they were much more likely to become paralyzed or even die.

Soon the disease began to spread.

And the polio virus didn't just spread disease. It also spread fear. Polio only struck during the summer and by 1915, when the disease infected thousands, warm weather and vacations were looked at with dread. For a long time, it looked like summers of fear were going to be a part of American life.

Polio did not discriminate. It infected black and white, rich and poor. It counted among its victims a wealthy future president.

It would take a child of the twentieth century to change all that. He would solve the riddle to one of the most tragic mysteries in the last one hundred years. Born to immigrant parents with little money, he was the first in his family to go to college. He would grow up to challenge some of the brightest men of his time. He would confront doctors and scientists who doubted his methods, questioned his abilities and ridiculed his results.

This is the story of the man who conquered one of the most frightening diseases in the twentieth century. This is the story of Jonas Salk.

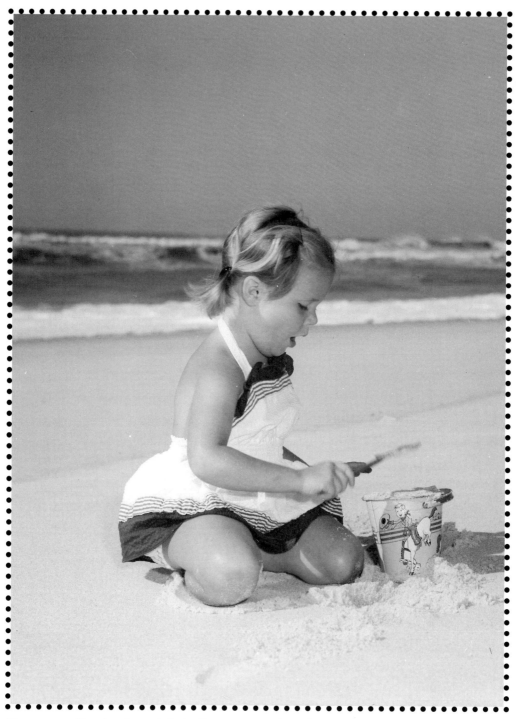

Because polio struck mainly in the summer, beaches like this one were often deserted during the epidemic.

Chapter 2
An Ambitious Childhood

• •

For hundreds of years, New York City has been the first step toward realizing the American dream. From the time when its streets were cobblestone and its name was New Amsterdam to the present day, it has represented the hopes and dreams for generations of immigrants.

Dolly and Daniel Salk were Russian Jews. Like many other people, they came to the United States hoping for a better life. Settling in the Lower East Side of Manhattan, they endured a difficult and crime-ridden neighborhood. They both worked in the garment industry. Daniel did some clothing design and manufacturing, while Dolly worked in sewing.

When Dolly became pregnant, the two saved until they could afford to move to a tenement, a low-rent, poorly maintained apartment in East Harlem.

Their first son, Jonas Edward Salk, was born on October 28, 1914. Although their new place was larger, the conditions were not much better than the Lower East Side. Perhaps that's why Jonas Salk's first words were "dirt, dirt."

Before Jonas enrolled in elementary school, the family moved to the Crotona section of the Bronx, a New York City borough across the East River from Manhattan. The new neighborhood was more middle-class, filled primarily with ambitious Jewish immigrants like the Salks.

There would be two other children, both boys: Herman and Lee.

Like many parents, the Salks wanted the best for their children. Dolly knew that in order for her sons to succeed in the world they needed to get a good education. Jonas' father had dropped out in high school, and his mother never even went to school.

In 1991, Jonas told an interviewer with the American Academy of Achievement that his mother was very ambitious for her children, even though the family didn't have much money. She wanted them to have more than she had, so she invested her life through her children.

"I was the eldest of three sons and the favorite and the one who had all of her attention, certainly until my little brother was born—I was about five years old then—and my youngest brother when I was about twelve. I was essentially an only child in the sense of having her interest and concerns and attention," Jonas recalled.

Although Dolly encouraged all her children to succeed academically (Herman would go on to become a veterinarian and Lee a clinical psychologist) Jonas was the one who received the most pressure. No matter how well he did in school, no matter how high his grades, his mother always expected him to do better.

Jonas rose to the challenge.

He was an extremely studious child. By the time he was in grade school, his nearsightedness required thick glasses; he was very thin and small for his age. In many ways, he was the type of kid who might have been picked on by bigger students.

This stopped being an issue when twelve-year-old Jonas was admitted to the very selective Townsend Harris High School. A public school, it was free and very challenging. Jonas was surrounded by children much like himself—very bright, hard-working and ambitious.

Salk wasn't just intelligent. He was also very empathetic. This means he deeply felt other people's pain and suffering. Growing up in the early 1900s, he witnessed first-hand the ravages of polio. Every summer, he'd notice the polio victims in his neighborhood. He would see the sick children his age—in wheelchairs or on crutches—who would never get better, who would never walk again. Jonas would see these children every day, and his heart would break a little.

Over eighty years ago, living in New York City during the summer was a very unpleasant experience. The heat would shimmer off the pavement in waves. There was no air conditioning. Since polio was believed to be contagious—spread through contact like the cold or flu—officials closed the public swimming pools and beaches were empty. Many parents, worried about the disease getting into their house, shut the windows tightly despite the temperatures.

Children who got polio would often be taken from their parents by the police, so they could be isolated in a hospital and not infect anyone else.

It was difficult to leave the city. Residents who wanted to get out of town were required to first see a doctor and get a certificate verifying they didn't have polio. Even then, traveling wasn't easy. At some small towns in upstate New York, townspeople would turn away travelers from the city at gunpoint.

It was impossible to grow up in the early part of the twentieth century and not be affected by polio.

Despite its impact, polio wasn't the only tragedy in America. In 1929, the month Jonas turned fifteen, the stock market crashed. People who had been worth millions of dollars were suddenly broke. Large companies went out of business, banks shut down. Unemployment rose to 25% and the homeless population exploded.

This period of time became known as the Great Depression. Jonas thought that by becoming a lawyer, he could help people with some of the problems that the Depression caused.

As a motivated student, he finished high school in only three years. However, despite his academic gifts, his options were more limited than some of his peers. There would be no expensive Ivy League college education in his future. Instead, Salk was admitted to the free City College of New York.

"My mother didn't think I would make a very good lawyer," Salk said in a 1991 interview, "probably because I could never win an argument with her. This change took place between leaving high school and entering college. I entered college enrolled as a pre-law student, but I changed to pre-med after I went through some soul searching."

Salk loved to unravel a mystery. He was the type of person who would keep working at a problem until he got it right. He also liked working alone; he had little interest in being supervised or having to answer to someone at every turn. Someone who likes being by himself and likes thinking alone is often called an introvert. Jonas Salk was definitely an introvert.

An old friend told Salk biographer Richard Carter that Jonas "was awfully difficult to know well. You somehow got the sense that perhaps he was holding back, not out of plain fear but because he was preoccupied with something."

14

Salk realized he didn't want to be a lawyer anymore. He wanted to become a doctor. However, he didn't want to be the type of doctor who treats patients or performs operations. He wanted to become a medical scientist. By digging into what caused disease, Salk hoped that his love for solving riddles would someday translate into helping other people. It was the perfect path for the times.

Around him, polio was still raging across the country like a violent hurricane. In 1916, it had infected over nine thousand people in New York City, killing nearly a third. By 1934, the year Salk earned his Bachelor of Science Degree from City College of New York, the disease even struck hospital workers in Los Angeles. Before the summer was over, nearly 5% of them were infected by polio. When Salk was accepted at the New York University School of Medicine, the risk of contracting polio was one all doctors faced.

Polio had become an epidemic—a disease that spreads from person to person, until it infects many people in a population. There was some talk about another, even deadlier epidemic—the Black Plague. That disease ravaged Europe during the Middle Ages and claimed nearly 25% of the population before subsiding.

Polio wasn't that dangerous yet. Except like the victims of the plague five hundred years before, no one knew exactly what caused polio. And no one knew how to prevent it.

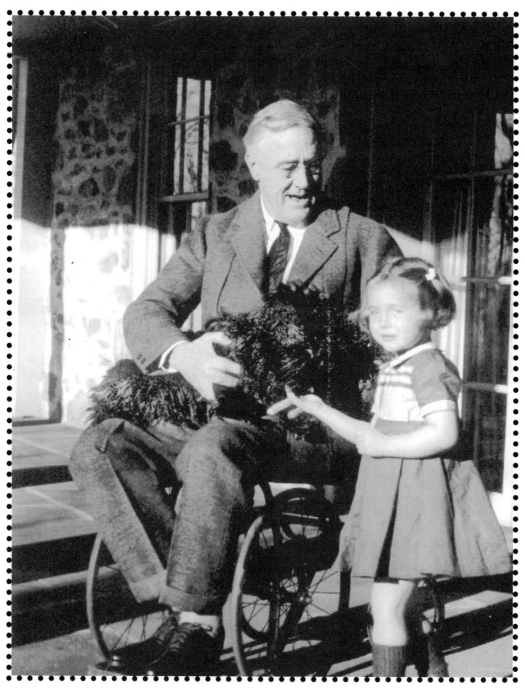

Proving that even the rich and the famous were not immune from the disease, polio struck wealthy Franklin Delano Roosevelt as a young man. Suffering permanent paralysis, he went on to be a tireless activist for the disease's cure and a popular president from 1933-1945.

Chapter 3
Polio Changes a Happy Life Forever

. . . .

F ranklin Delano Roosevelt enjoyed a life that many people envied. He was an attractive young man, born into a wealthy family. He ran as the Democratic vice-presidential candidate in 1920. Even though his party lost the election, he'd gained enough attention that people were talking about him being president someday. His name was in the newspapers: in society columns and on the front pages.

In the summer of 1921, Roosevelt took a well-deserved vacation. His happy life was changed forever. It didn't matter that he was rich, or that he might one day be president.

He got polio. The disease would permanently damage his legs—he would never walk again. Roosevelt would spend the rest of his life in a wheelchair. The disease would make him an activist.

The sad reality is that in many cases, dangerous diseases are often ignored until they strike down the rich or the famous. In the 1980s, Acquired Immune Deficiency Syndrome (AIDS) wasn't given much attention until it struck people like actor Rock Hudson, musician Liberace, and basketball player Magic Johnson.

Polio had been a well-known and greatly feared disease long before it infected Roosevelt. Because he was a man with political connections and access to money, polio treatment became well-funded when he put his talents behind eliminating the deadly disease.

Roosevelt enlisted the aid of his law firm partner, Basil O'Conner. A man who'd grown up poor, he put himself through Dartmouth College and went on to law school at Harvard. As a lawyer, O'Conner was rich by the time he was thirty-two and became Roosevelt's business partner.

The two often met at the Meriwether Inn in Warm Springs, Georgia. Roosevelt believed the warm water in the pools would help his legs recover. He believed other polio patients would benefit from the treatment as well and decided to buy the inn for them.

"I thought he was crazy," O'Conner told Salk biographer Richard Carter. "I couldn't have been less interested in the project."

Despite his partner's misgivings, Roosevelt and some friends purchased the Meriwether for $200,000 in 1926. They began the Warm Springs Polio Foundation for victims of polio and opened the inn's doors to anyone, regardless of their ability to pay.

In 1928, Roosevelt became governor of New York state. O'Conner recalled that Roosevelt told him, "Take over Warm Springs, old fella: you're in."

O'Conner added, "I tell you, I had no desire to be 'in.' I was never a public do-gooder and had no aspirations of that kind. But I started enjoying it."

In 1932, Roosevelt was elected president of the United States. The next year, Carl Byoir, a public relations expert, suggested that dances be held across the country in honor of the new president's birthday. The money raised would go to the Warm Springs Polio Foundation.

In 1934, over 6,000 dances in 4,300 communities across the United States raised more than one million dollars. Following the event, Roosevelt spoke to the nation on the largest radio broadcast in history. "As a representative of the hundreds of thousands of crippled children in our country," he said, "the next step would be to spread the gospel for the care and cure of crippled children in every part of this kindly land to enable us to make the same relative progress as we have made in the field of tuberculosis."

Thanks to the success of medical research, the disease of tuberculosis—which had killed many people in the nineteenth and early twentieth centuries—was slowly being eradicated.

The appeal for similar efforts for polio could have been directed to Jonas Salk, who had just begun medical school. His fellow students considered him an odd fit. Most of them wanted to become surgeons or other kinds of doctors who deal directly with patients. But Salk's dream was to become a medical researcher, a scientist. His peers didn't think he had the creativity to succeed in that field.

Salk said in a 1991 interview with the American Academy of Achievement that "I would say that I spent more time alone than I did in social settings." This tendency to prefer his own company was one reason he made little impression on other medical students.

However, at least one of his professors was very impressed by Salk.

"The professor of chemistry, Dr. R. Keith Cannon, tapped me on the shoulder and asked me to come and see him," Salk recalled in the 1991 interview. "I was quite sure that he was going to tell me that I was failing and give me some bad news. Instead of which, he offered me an opportunity to drop out for a year and work with him in chemistry."

Salk leaped at the chance. For the next year he learned techniques in protein chemistry which would later help him solve the riddles of polio.

Returning to school in 1936, Salk quickly began to make his mark. He published his first scientific paper, an unusual accomplishment for a second-year medical student. He also began to question the popular medical opinions of his time—an important step to becoming a scientist.

"The first moment that a question occurred to me that did influence my future career, occurred in my second year of medical school," Salk told an interviewer with the American Academy of Achievement in 1991.

A professor had explained how toxins which were chemically treated could be given to immunize a patient against tetanus. By giving someone an injection of "killed" tetanus, the patient would be protected against the disease.

"The following lecture," Salk recalled in the interview, "we were told that for immunization against a virus disease, you have to experience the infection and you could not induce immunity with so-called 'killed' or inactivated, chemically treated virus preparation. Well, somehow, that struck me. What struck me was that both statements couldn't be true."

In his last year as a medical student, Salk was recruited to work with a well-known scientist, Dr. Thomas Francis Jr., who had discovered the type-B influenza virus.

"I spent the first month learning to take out the lungs of infected mice, and extract the influenza virus from them," Salk related to his biographer. "It was excellent preparation for later studies and ideas."

By then Salk's ideas about "killed" versus "live" vaccines were thoughts he probably focused on influenza—the flu. An earlier pair of experiments with possible polio vaccines had resulted in tragedy. One of the experiments was conducted by a doctor at New York University, the school Salk attended.

In 1935, two types of vaccines for polio had been tested on people. One had the "killed" virus, the other was a "living" version. Over twelve thousand children received one of the vaccines. Following the shots, six of those children died and three were paralyzed. Not only did it kill people, the vaccine didn't prevent polio.

Under the direction of Basil O'Conner, the newly formed National Foundation for Infantile Paralysis—polio was also known as infantile paralysis—decided not to move forward with the testing of any more vaccines until a great deal more research was done. For Jonas Salk, the future lay not in polio, but in the flu.

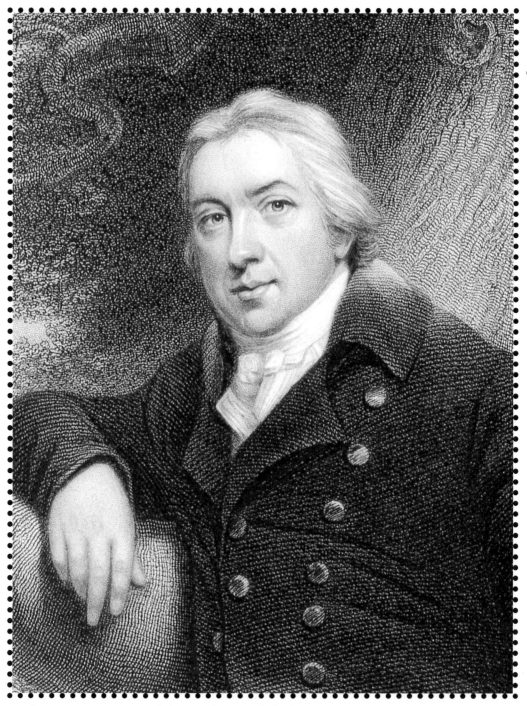

Modern vaccination can be traced to English doctor Edward Jenner, whose discovery in 1796 that injections of cowpox prevented smallpox saved thousands of lives.

Chapter 4
The War Against the Flu

It would take a celebrity to come up with the idea which would provide much of the funding for polio research. "We could ask the people to send their dimes directly to the White House," actor-singer Eddie Cantor said during a speech at the MGM movie studio lot. "Think about the thrill the people would get... and we could call it, The March of Dimes!"

From 1938, when 2.7 million dimes were mailed directly to the White House, to 1955 when the March of Dimes earned the National Foundation for Infantile Paralysis 67 million dollars, never before had so many private citizens contributed directly to eliminate a dreaded disease.

In the beginning, most of the money went towards treatments—everything from hot springs and warm wraps to physical therapy. Later on it would provide thousands of iron lungs, frightening contraptions which basically did the breathing for paralyzed polio victims.

Yet initially, little money was spent on research.

"Why do we use all that dough to dip [polio victims] in warm water?" asked Paul De Kruif, a famous scientist. He reportedly told the manager of the Warm Springs resort, "That doesn't cure them any more than it cured Roosevelt. Why don't you ask the President to devote part of that big dough to research on polio prevention?"

President Roosevelt listened to this plea. Each year, more and more scientists were enlisted in this effort. But Jonas Salk was not one of them.

He celebrated his graduation from medical school in 1939 by getting married to Donna Lindsay, a psychology major at Smith College. She told Salk biographer Richard Carter that "There was no shell in evidence when I met him. He was a good dancer, an amusing and exciting conversationalist and as different from the stereotype of the one-track scientist as anyone possibly could be."

Lindsay was the daughter of a very successful dentist, and some of her friends wondered why she was marrying the child of a garment worker. Despite those questions, Donna loved Salk, and believed in his future. As later events would prove, she had good reason to.

Salk applied for an internship at Mount Sinai Hospital in New York. Although he was competing against 250 other top-ranked medical school graduates, he was one of a dozen who were selected for the position.

The job was unpaid—in the beginning Salk's wife supported them both. After a year, when he gained residency, Salk would finally get a paycheck—fifteen dollars a month!

Jonas Salk's empathy served him well in his new job. "It's no injustice to anyone to say that he was the best intern in the hospital," one physician who remembered Salk said in an anonymous interview. The doctor went on to tell biographer Richard Carter that Salk was "as versatile and promising a physician as any of them—and by far the most mature and reliable."

Although he was only 25, Salk was respected by his peers, even being elected president of the house staff. One prominent surgeon offered Salk a job. Although his mother Dolly begged him to take it—the position would offer both a stable salary and prestige—Salk turned it down. He knew what he wanted to do with his life.

Salk had decided to become a virologist, a scientist who studies viruses and how they behave. This was a very new field and a difficult one. Viruses were considerably smaller than bacteria—one million viruses together would cover a surface less than an inch long. In fact, until the 1940s there wouldn't even be microscopes powerful enough to see them. Viruses were also notoriously difficult to work with. Poliomyelitis—the virus responsible for polio—couldn't be grown in a test tube or a petri dish. It could only be kept alive in human beings or in monkeys.

Despite the challenges, Salk was fascinated by this infant field. He knew it would be filled with both the complex riddles and the opportunities to help people that he craved. As his residency at Mount Sinai drew to a close, Salk began applying to numerous medical foundations to study viruses. One after another turned him down.

According to some reports, at least one foundation refused to even consider Salk because he was Jewish. At this time anti-Semitism—or prejudice against Jews—was very common in the medical establishment. Across the ocean, in Europe, Adolph Hitler and Nazi Germany were responsible for the eventual annihilation of millions of Jewish people during World War II. Yet back in the United States—which still hadn't entered the war—many people sympathized with at least some of Hitler's philosophy.

Questions about whether or not America should be involved in the growing conflict overseas effectively ended on December 7, 1941. On that date, the Japanese attacked Pearl Harbor, a military base in Hawaii. As the United States joined the war, Jonas Salk was offered the opportunity that would change his life forever.

"There are two tragedies in life," Jonas Salk said. "One is to not get what you want; the other is to get what you want." What Salk wanted was a research appointment to one of the many foundations in and around New York City. What he got was an invitation from Dr. Francis to move to the University of Michigan and work on the influenza vaccine.

Salk had worked with Francis while he was in medical school and greatly admired the man. Although Salk was very interested in viruses, he'd never considered working with vaccines. Yet the work Francis was proposing they do was very important to the war effort.

In 1918, a flu epidemic had killed 850,000 Americans, 44,000 of whom were soldiers. Because of the way soldiers must live in close contact with one another in often difficult conditions, viruses like the flu can be spread quickly. Francis hoped to discover a vaccine to save them. Salk decided to join him.

In 1942, Salk and his wife Dolly moved to Ann Arbor, Michigan, where the university was located. It was a very different situation for a city boy who'd lived in New York his whole life. Ann Arbor was a pleasant college town, and the rural farmhouse the Salks moved into relied on a wood-burning stove for cooking and heating. Salk enjoyed the change.

In the laboratories of the University of Michigan, Salk labored with Francis to find a vaccine to prevent influenza. It was also Salk's first contact with the National Foundation for Infantile Paralysis. Although none of Salk's work at this point would involve polio, the organization was funding the research because they felt flu vaccines could lead to the development of polio vaccines.

In many ways, vaccines offer protection from a disease by using the disease itself. By swallowing or being injected with a milder form of a dangerous disease, people who are vaccinated are protected from the illness.

One of the first groups of people to practice this form of medicine were Middle Eastern women who would scrape off the sores of a person infected with smallpox and inject the substance into healthy people. This crude method actually worked: those treated that way usually didn't get smallpox.

Unfortunately in order to be protected from smallpox—a potentially deadly disease—someone else always had to get it.

In 1796 that changed.

An English doctor named Edward Jenner had noticed milkmaids coming into contact with "cowpox" from sores on a cow's udder. After this contact, these milkmaids didn't get smallpox. Jenner engaged in a risky experiment.

He scraped off some of the cowpox and injected it into an eight-year-old boy. As expected, the boy got sick, but he recovered. Six weeks later, the doctor injected the same boy with smallpox sores. The boy stayed healthy— he was now immune to smallpox.

In 1798, Jenner injected hundreds of people with cowpox during a devastating smallpox epidemic. The people he injected became immune to the disease. In a book he wrote on the subject, Jenner called the technique "vaccination." The word comes from the Latin word "vacca," which means cow. Although current vaccinations don't involve cows, the term is still used to describe the procedure.

One hundred and fifty years later, doctors had developed vaccinations for all kinds of illnesses. Unfortunately, vaccinations for most viruses didn't work. One reason is that viruses like those for polio or the flu have several different types, or strains. Protection from one strain doesn't mean a person is protected from another. Also, because viruses attach themselves to healthy cells, killing the virus sometimes involves killing healthy cells, which further endangers the patient.

Still another problem was when a live version of the polio or flu virus was injected into a healthy patient, it could develop into a full-blown version of the disease. This is what happened in 1935 when several children got polio from an experimental vaccine.

Salk and Francis believed the solution was to use killed versions of the virus. Salk noticed how antibodies— the body's natural defense against viruses—developed even with a killed vaccine. Salk worked hard to develop a test to study how much the antibody levels in the blood stream were raised by a virus. If antibody levels increased sufficiently, the vaccine of killed virus would be effective. Salk was widely credited with developing the test to determine the level of antibodies in the blood.

By the time Salk and Francis began research on a flu vaccine, veterinarians had already successfully attempted injecting killed viruses into animals. By using a chemical called formalin on the virus, its destructive abilities were reduced. The body, however, would respond as if the virus was at full strength. Antibody levels would go up and the patient would become immune.

The Ann Arbor researchers tested their theory by vaccinating both college students and soldiers. In one test during the winter of 1943-1944, 2,500 soldiers were given injections. Half of the men received an injection of the actual vaccine, half received what is called a placebo, or a "fake" vaccine. Among the soldiers who received the flu vaccine, there was a 75% lower rate of flu infection. The vaccine worked!

After World War II ended, Salk wanted the chance to test his theories about vaccinations. Although he'd enjoyed his time at Ann Arbor, by 1947 Salk was ready to be in charge. Once again, he needed someone to believe in him.

World War II was over. The attentions of the American people and their government turned closer to home, to a battle which had still many casualties and no clear end in sight: the war against polio.

Already the disease had lost its greatest activist. Franklin Delano Roosevelt died on April 12, 1945, at the Warm Springs, Georgia retreat he'd bought for polio victims nearly twenty-five years earlier. Despite the loss, Basil O'Conner, Roosevelt's long-time business partner, continued his tireless crusade against the disease.

In the late 1940s, the news was not good. Although the disease now claimed over thirty thousand victims annually, scientists had abandoned the idea of finding a vaccine for polio. Ever since the tragic vaccine experiments of 1935, scientists felt polio was more likely to be prevented or treated by a new drug. Worse, the various groups of scientists involved with the quest were being pulled apart by arguments over everything from who should get credit to the methods that they were pursuing.

In Ann Arbor, Michigan, Jonas Salk was engaged in a war of his own. He'd been working at the school since 1942, and after the war ended he realized he was never going to get the kind of scientific freedom he desired. Although his professional relationship with Dr. Thomas Francis Jr. was still decent, Jonas wanted to conduct his own research on viruses.

Salk applied to work at viral labs across the country, from the University of California to Western Reserve in Cleveland, Ohio. He even applied to his former employer, Mount Sinai Hospital in New York.

But despite the groundbreaking work he'd done in developing a flu vaccine, they all turned him down. Back home in New York City, his mother Dolly pleaded with her son to move back and start a private practice. She believed it would be the best way for Jonas to support his growing family, which now included two young sons, Peter and Daniel.

Jonas refused to consider private practice. He wanted to be in research. After he spent months searching for an opportunity, the University of Pittsburgh finally gave him a chance. They invited him to tour the school and consider a job as director of virus research.

The school wasn't exactly a top research facility.

"The medical school had a grant of about $1,800 from the American Society for the Study of High Blood Pressure," a former faculty member recalled. "I think that was the entire research program. Furthermore, the place was filthy."

"Tommy Francis thought I was making a mistake," Salk told biographer Richard Carter. "I can remember someone asking me, 'What's in Pittsburgh, for heaven's sake?' And I answered, 'I guess I fell in love.' What I was in love with, of course, was the prospect of independence."

Only after Jonas Salk moved his family to unfamiliar Pittsburgh in October of 1947, did he realize how far his dreams for independence were from reality. For one thing, when he'd toured the school he'd been told the nearby Municipal Hospital would also be available to him. It wasn't. Second, his lab space turned out to be a cramped and dusty basement. Although the dean of the medical school who'd hired him, Dr. William S. McEllroy, promised to help Salk, his power was limited. Salk had to fight for every extra inch of space he got.

Worse, the promised independence was an illusion as well. The school already had a virus researcher—Dr. Max A. Lauffer. Although the scientist had gained attention for his work with viruses which attack plants, he didn't share Salk's interest in animal viruses. Because Salk had to answer to Lauffer, the two men clashed repeatedly.

Once again, the National Foundation for Infantile Paralysis helped Jonas in an unexpected way.

From before the 1900s, strides had been made in polio research.

In 1898, Dutch scientist Martinus Beijerinck discovered viruses. In 1908, Karl Landsteiner proved polio fit into this category of "intracellular microbes," which enter the insides of living cells and use their proteins and other genetic material to reproduce, usually killing or damaging the healthy cell in the process.

The work of Australian virologist Sir Macfarlane Burnet in 1933 concluded that there were numerous strains of polioviruses. While Salk had been at Ann Arbor, scientists were making progress in identifying the causes of polio. Unfortunately, by 1947, a treatment had not yet been discovered.

As Salk was struggling to gain independence and lab space, Harry Weaver began working as research director for the National Foundation for Infantile Paralysis.

Weaver had a problem. Unlike many scientists, Weaver believed a vaccine would eventually prevent polio. Still, he realized that one of the biggest challenges to finding a vaccine lay in the variety of strains. Although it was known that there was more than one strain—or type—of polio, no one was sure how many different strains there were. This was critical. If a vaccine protected against two different strains, someone might get the shot and still catch polio from a third strain.

Unfortunately, identifying all the strains of polio would be a costly, time-consuming project. Worse, it would require an experienced virologist to oversee it, but because of the drudgery and unstimulating nature of the job, few virologists would be interested.

Weaver knew about Salk's work with flu vaccines, and quickly found out the doctor was at the University of Pittsburgh, fighting for lab space and independence. In late 1947, Weaver and O'Conner met with Salk and several others at the university to see if they would be interested in the project. Salk, who'd been laboring in cramped quarters with little money, knew it would be the chance he needed. For the University of Pittsburgh, the project would mean a chance to improve the school's shoddy reputation.

It would be an enormous undertaking. Pittsburgh would be joined by universities in Southern California, Kansas and Utah. The project was expected to consume two to three years, millions of dollars and many monkeys.

Still, after he met with Salk, Weaver knew the doctor was perfect for the task. He felt Jonas Salk would be "perfectly comfortable with the idea of using hundreds of monkeys and running dozens of experiments at a time," Weaver later told an interviewer. "Jonas could accept the possibility that so many old-timers could not, that regardless of prior theory, you might be able to immunize human beings against polio if you put antibody into their blood."

Salk and the university received an initial grant of $250,000 from the National Foundation. Before his work was completed, Salk's research would require over $1,250,000 and nearly 30,000 monkeys.

Salk was ready to get to work identifying the different types of the poliovirus. Unfortunately he immediately ran into conflict.

At a virus typing committee meeting on January 14, 1948, he listened as other, more experienced scientists told him how to conduct the study. They wanted him to start by infecting monkeys with known polio strains and then add unknown viruses to the animals.

Salk believed this was a waste of time and he let the scientists know it. He felt it would be faster—and just as effective—to inject the uninfected monkeys with only unknown strains of the polio virus. Then he could test the antibody level in the monkeys' blood. Similar to work he'd already done with the flu virus at Ann Arbor, the advantage was that even if the strain he injected was too weak to cause an infection, there would still be new antibodies in the blood.

When he asked the other doctors why they didn't consider this, Salk told biographer Richard Carter that

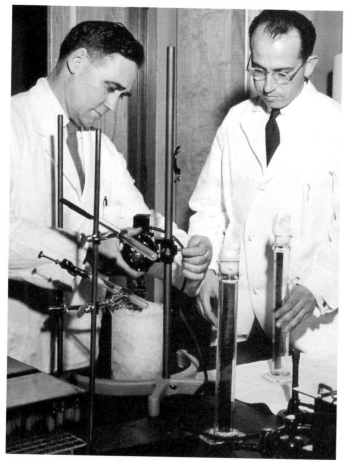

Jonas Salk helped turn the University of Pittsburgh into a top facility for polio research despite its poor reputation.

"Albert Sabin sat back and turned to me and said, 'You should know better than to ask a question like that!' It was like being kicked in the teeth."

Albert Sabin was a Russian doctor who, in 1936, proved polioviruses grow in the upper digestive tract. His opinion was considered more important than Salk's.

Salk didn't become discouraged when the committee insisted he do it their way. He just followed their orders and did his own experiments at night.

"The typing program was to take three years," Salk told Carter, "but our laboratory had the whole thing solved before the end of the first year. Everything that happened during the last two years was merely confirmatory. What could I do? I couldn't slap those people in the face and call them dumb bunnies."

Meanwhile, other breakthroughs were occurring.

In 1948, Dr. Robert Green, a professor of bacteriology at the University of Minnesota, implanted bits of human intestinal membrane in rabbits' eyes. When he added a polio virus, it multiplied quickly, proving that polio could grow in tissue that wasn't from the nervous system.

The next year, Drs. John Enders, Fred Robbins and Tom Weller demonstrated a technique to grow poliovirus without using monkeys.

These two discoveries were very important. Viruses grown in nervous tissue had caused severe—sometimes even fatal—allergic reactions when used as a vaccine. Also, growing poliovirus without relying on monkeys would eliminate a tremendous amount of both expense and difficulty.

Jonas Salk believed he and his team were ready. In July of 1950, he asked the National Foundation for Infantile Paralysis if he could begin researching a new polio vaccine.

If the country had ever needed polio prevention, it was in the 1950s. Every summer, more than 30,000 new cases of polio were reported. Tragically, Basil O'Conner—a tireless crusader against the virus for nearly three decades—had to face the disease in his own family. His adult daughter, Bettyann O'Conner Culver, was infected. Although she recovered, she would suffer from some paralysis for the rest of her life.

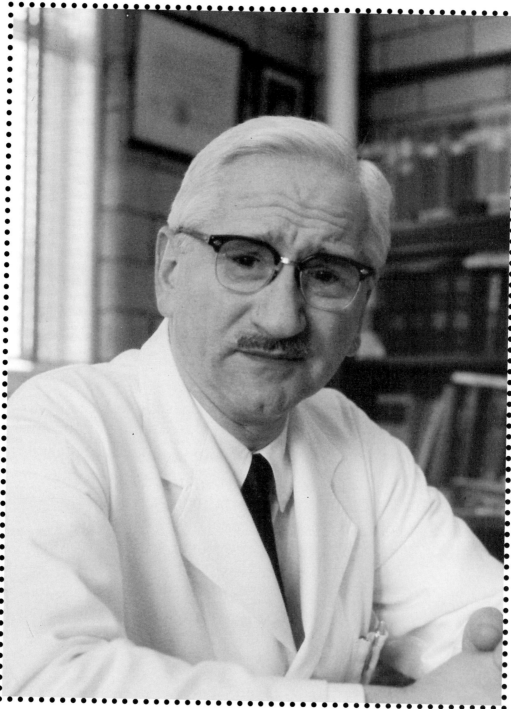

Dr. Albert Sabin gained fame for his work in helping to solve the polio riddle. He developed a widely used vaccine several years after Salk.

Chapter 5

Vaccine!

·····································

Whenever Jonas Salk or a member of his team needed a reminder of their work's importance, they only needed to climb a few stairs. From his early days at the University of Pittsburgh, struggling in a cramped basement, Salk had taken over a large lab at the nearby Municipal Hospital. Just a few stories overhead was the polio ward. It wasn't uncommon for a dozen new patients to be admitted each night during the summer months.

Salk was given approval in 1951 to work on a new vaccine, but he still encountered resistance. The reason was because he believed the best way to safely prevent polio was with a killed virus.

Once again, Salk was opposed by Dr. Albert Sabin. Sabin was working on his own vaccine—using a live virus— and he argued that even if Salk's vaccine worked, it would take at least fifteen years before it was ready.

"The principle that I tried to establish," Salk explained in an interview with the American Academy of Achievement, "was that it was not really necessary to run the risk of infection, which would have been the case if one were to try to develop an attenuated or weakened polio virus vaccine. It seemed to me the safer and more certain way to proceed; if we could inactivate the virus, we could move on to a vaccine very quickly."

With his goal clear in his mind, Salk returned to the University of Pittsburgh's virus research laboratory. In addition to directing that operation, Salk had also been promoted to full professor of bacteriology.

As he worked to develop a vaccine, his greatest problem was duplicating the work of Dr. Enders' team. No matter how hard he tried, he couldn't grow the poliovirus the same way they had. Salk's philosophy about the worst thing is getting what you want proved true again.

In the Pittsburgh team's initial failure to replicate Enders' results, they managed to discover the most antigenic viruses—polioviruses with the highest antibodies. They found three strains—one of each type—that were strong, stable and reliable.

They were perfect for the vaccine.

As they worked to cultivate this poliovirus, Salk continued to learn from other scientists' recent discoveries. In March of 1951, he attended a lecture given by Dr. Isabel Morgan Mountain. He learned how she'd successfully killed polio viruses in a solution of formalin, a form of the lab chemical formaldehyde.

After injecting monkeys with the killed virus solution, Dr. Mountain learned their antibody levels rose to the same level as if they been injected with live virus.

Dr. Salk contributed his own findings. He'd discovered that when mineral oil was added to his vaccine it produced more antibodies in the monkeys.

Armed with new information from the lecture, Salk returned to the lab. Using kidney tissue from monkeys, the researchers tested combinations of all three types of polio strains. They then experimented with different levels of formalin at different temperatures. Using the vaccine—made up of mineral oil, formalin, and all three strong strains of poliovirus—Salk and the other researchers injected the killed virus into infected monkeys.

The vaccine worked; the level of antibodies increased.

In December of 1951, Salk presented his results to the Immunization Committee. The members were worried that there might still be live virus present in Salk's vaccine despite all of his precautions. If that happened, the tragedy of 1935 could be repeated.

Although Sabin was opposed to the vaccine, in the end the committee decided the best way to test Salk's new vaccine was on children already infected with polio. Their antibodies would be tested after the injection to determine if the antibody levels rose.

In 1952, Drs. Dorothy Hartsmann and David Brodie proved polio entered the bloodstream after first being in the digestive tract. A week to a month later, the virus would reach the nervous system.

This was critical information. It meant antibodies in the blood could create a wall between the poliovirus and the nervous system—safely preventing paralysis. Salk knew he was close. He started working sixteen-hour days as he tirelessly oversaw the creation of a killed poliovirus vaccine.

In the spring of 1952, Salk prepared to test his vaccine on children infected with polio. He traveled to the D.T. Watson Home for Crippled Children. The doctors allowed Salk to test the vaccine on 79 young patients. Because of their polio infection, the children already had a certain level of immunity. By testing the antibody's increase after the injection, Salk would be able to see if the vaccine was effective.

A nurse would later say Salk was "obviously not just a scientist on an experiment but a man deeply concerned about the human importance of the experiment."

Salk barely slept. He wasn't just worried about whether or not his vaccine failed. He was worried about the children's safety.

His worries were unnecessary. None of the children got sick. Just as importantly, the injection had raised antibodies in every child who received the killed virus vaccine. Some of the children got a placebo or fake vaccine; they showed no results.

The vaccine worked!

As Salk continued his research, the summer of 1952 was a reminder of how important a vaccine was. The epidemic exploded. Instead of 25,000 new polio infections there would be over 50,000. One out of every four infected was an adult.

In a January 1953 meeting of the Immunization Committee, Dr. Sabin again expressed his doubts about the safety of Salk's vaccine. Besides, Sabin said again, it would take fifteen years for Salk's version to be ready. Sabin promised his own live virus vaccine would be available much sooner.

This time, the committee listened to Salk. In 1953, the whole nation would also listen.

In February, *Time* magazine ran a piece on the vaccine with Salk's picture. Although the doctor wrote an article about his progress for the respected *Journal of the American Medical Association*, he got more attention from an article by New York gossip columnist Earl Wilson.

Worried the public was relying on inaccurate information, Salk agreed to speak to the country on a radio broadcast. On March 26, 1953, Basil O'Conner introduced the researcher by saying, "You, the American people have characteristically made yourself active partners—stockholders, if you will—in finding a polio vaccine."

Salk then explained in clear language exactly where he was with the vaccine. Scientists were notoriously difficult to interview because they relied on complicated terms and unfamiliar descriptions of experiments. Because he was so plain-spoken, Salk was an instant hit with both reporters and the public.

That spring, Salk began the most crucial part of his study, by testing the polio vaccine on people who'd never had the disease. He tested the first batch on himself, and his wife Donna, along with his now nine-year-old son Peter and six-year-old Daniel. Worried that the needle would scare his youngest son, Salk tested the vaccine on three-year-old Jonathon while the toddler slept.

"When you engage in human experimentation," Salk said, "you must proceed in a somewhat cautious manner and be prepared for the unforeseen and the unknowable."

When Salk's family showed increased antibodies but no ill effects from the vaccine, the doctor began field trials. From 5,000 children in Pittsburgh in 1953 to nearly two million in early 1954, Salk conducted his vaccination tests across 44 states. Some of the children received the real vaccine, some a placebo. Until the experiment was over, not even the scientist knew who was getting what.

These young people were "polio pioneers," the first to test a vaccine which could eliminate one of the most deadly diseases of the twentieth century.

"On April 12, 1955 the announcement was made of the field trial results in Ann Arbor by Dr. Francis, who had conducted the field trial," Salk remembered in a 1991 interview. "He was my mentor... This was a very public event

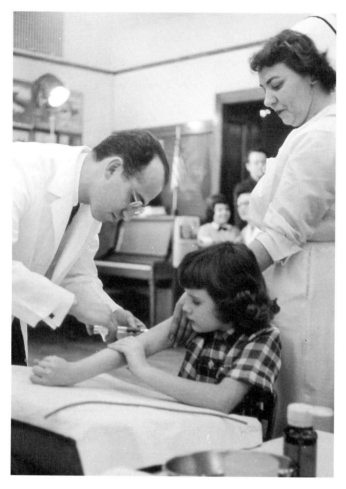
With careful aim and a gentle touch, Dr. Salk injects his vaccine.

and it was done with great fanfare. Many people were invited; scientists and non-scientists... I felt myself very much in the eye of the hurricane, because all this swirling was going on. It was at that moment that everything changed."

It was at that moment that the world learned Salk's vaccine would indeed prevent polio.

By 1956 thirty million people had been vaccinated; by 1957 fifty percent of all Americans under age 50 had received the necessary three injections of Salk's vaccine for total immunity. Polio rates dropped from over thirty-eight thousand infections in 1954 to less than one thousand by 1962.

Jonas Salk was a hero to the American public, as famous as any movie star and much more important. Still, even his discovery didn't eliminate conflict. The American

Medical Association fought with the doctor because the polio vaccine was being given away for free. Salk not only insisted on this, but didn't even patent the vaccine—although he could have made millions from the vaccine, he chose instead to give it away.

He was nominated for the Nobel Prize for Medicine, one of the highest honors a doctor can receive, but he did not get the prize. Many felt this was because instead of discovering a brand-new vaccine, Salk had created the killed poliovirus using other scientists' techniques.

Dr. Albert Sabin agreed with this point of view. Although Sabin was pushed into the shadows by Salk's achievement, when Sabin's live poliovirus vaccine was ready, the AMA approved it before it was released, something they'd never done before. Because it could be swallowed once on a lump of sugar and didn't require any injections, the Sabin vaccine quickly became more popular in the United States than Salk's.

But because he was the first man to successfully vaccinate large numbers of people, Jonas Salk remains the person most commonly associated with the elimination of polio in this country.

In 1963, Salk used his prestige to found the Salk Institute for Biological Studies in La Jolla, California. He hoped to combine a variety of scientific disciplines in order to move forward in the prevention of diseases. In the 1960s and 70s, much of the institute's work was devoted to cancer research. In the eighties and nineties, its focus switched to the study of AIDS.

In 1968, Donna and Jonas Salk divorced. Two years later, he married French painter Francoise Gilot.

In 1987, a new, more potent inactivated form of the polio vaccine was created with greater antigenic content. Even so, at that time the most widely used method of innoculation remained the oral polio vaccine developed by Dr. Sabin. It was also rapidly becoming the only way to contract the disease. Though only a very small number of people actually got the disease each year from the live vaccine, Salk had always argued that no one should be at risk from the innoculation.

In 1995, still active in his work at the institute, Jonas Salk died of congestive heart failure. The controversy between the Salk vaccine and the Sabin vaccine did not die with him, however.

In 1997, the American Academy of Pediatrics proposed new methods of vaccination which included two killed (IPV) followed by two live (OPV) vaccinations. On June 16, 1999, the Centers for Disease Control in Atlanta, Georgia voted to eliminate use of Sabin's oral polio vaccine in favor of Salk's injected polio vaccine. By January 2000, only the injected form was recommended. As polio is now considered eradicated from the U.S. population, the oral polio vaccine is considered a greater risk than the threat of the disease from other sources.

In many ways Salk's medical legacy still lives on. The institute he founded continues to do groundbreaking research. Jonas's career also inspired his sons, as all three became doctors. Two of them are scientists, just like their father.

Jonas Salk Chronology

- 1914, is born in New York City.
- 1926, enters Townsend Harris Hall, a public high school for gifted students.
- 1929, enrolls in City College of New York as a pre-law student.
- 1934, receives Bachelor of Science degree from City College.
- 1934, is admitted to New York University School of Medicine.
- 1935, takes a year off from school to do advanced work in biochemistry.
- 1938, works with Dr. Thomas Francis Jr. on killed influenza viruses.
- 1939, receives his medical degree from New York University.
- 1940, becomes medical intern at Mount Sinai Hospital in New York.
- 1942, joins University of Michigan's School of Public Health in order to develop a safe flu vaccine.
- 1947, becomes head of Virus Research Lab at the University of Pittsburgh.
- 1952, inoculates first volunteers—including himself, his wife, and his three children—with polio vaccine.
- 1955, makes public the news of discovery of polio vaccine.
- 1963, founds Jonas Salk Institute for Biological Studies in La Jolla, California.
- 1980s/1990s, devotes much of his time as researcher to finding a cure for AIDS.
- 1995, dies of congestive heart failure.

Polio Timeline

3700 B.C. Ancient skeletons show signs of polio

400 B.C. Greek physician Hippocrates writes about a disease which causes paralysis.

1718 Using a technique brought back from the Middle East, Lady Mary Wortly Montagu uses sores from victims of mild smallpox to protect healthy people from the disease.

1789 Dr. Michael Underwood's book about childhood diseases describes a palsy which weakens limbs.

1796 Dr. Edward Jenner uses vaccinations of cowpox to prevent smallpox.

1877 Louis Pasteur learns to culture disease-causing organisms in order to develop vaccines.

1890s Working with anthrax, Robert Koch shows that a specific organism can cause a specific disease.

1890s Jacob Von Heine establishes that polio is not a form of palsy but a separate disease.

1898 Dutch scientist Martinus Beijerinck discovers viruses.

1908 Karl Landsteiner isolates the specific virus that causes polio.

1921 Future president Franklin Delano Roosevelt contracts polio during a family vacation, which leads to his activism for polio treatment and prevention.

1933 The work of Australian virologist Sir Macfarlane Burnet concludes that there were several strains of polioviruses.

1935 Experimental polio vaccines fail; six children die.

1936 Albert Sabin proves polioviruses grow in the upper digestive tract.

1948 Salk begins identifying various strains of poliovirus.

1948 Dr. Robert Green proves that polio could grow in tissue that wasn't from the nervous system.

1949 Drs. John Enders, Fred Robbins and Tom Weller demonstrate a technique to grow polio virus without using monkeys.

1951 Dr. Isabel Morgan Mountain proves formalin is effective in killing poliovirus.

1952 Drs. Dorothy Hartsmann and David Brodie prove polio enters the bloodstream after first being in the digestive tract; a week to a month later, the virus reaches the nervous system.

1952/1955 Salk conducts field trials of vaccine.

1955 Salk's killed poliovirus vaccine made available to the public.

1963 Sabin's live poliovirus vaccine becomes more popular in US than Salk's because it can be swallowed rather than injected

1997 CDC recommends that both the killed (IPV) vaccine and the live (OPV) vaccine be given: two doses of killed followed by two doses of live

2000 CDC recommends only the IPV (Salk vaccine) as polio is considered eradicated from the U.S.

Further Reading

On the web:

www.pbs.org - On the Edge - Paralyzing Polio
www.Achievement.Org - "American Academy of Achievement" - Interview
    with Jonas Salk
Netscape: Yahoo! Health - Disease, Condition or General Topics (Polio)

Young Adult:

Sherwood, Victoria. *Makers of Modern Science: Jonas Salk.* New York:
    Facts on File, 1993

Adult:

Carter, Richard. *Breakthrough: The Saga of Jonas Salk.* New York: Trident
    Press, 1966
Klein, Aaron E. *Trial By Fury: The Polio Vaccine Controversy.* New York:
    Scribner, 1972
Kriegel, Leonard. *The Long Walk Home.* New York: Appleton-Century, 1964
Rogers, Naomi. *Dirt and Disease: Polio Before FDR.* New Brunswick, N.J:
    Rutgers University Press, 1992
Smith, Jane S. *Patenting the Sun: Polio and the Salk Vaccine.* New York, W.
    Morrow, 1990

Glossary

antibody - protein produced by body as a response to viruses or bacteria.
antigen - substance which activates an antibody.
bacteria - one-celled organisms including parasites; some attack, some do
    not.
culture - the process of growing microbes in a laboratory.
epidemic - widespread outbreak of a disease.
electron microscope - powerful microscope which magnifies by using beam
    of electrons.
Formaldehyde - a strong disinfectant used to sterilize.
formalin - a solution made formaldehyde and water.
immunity - resistance to disease-causing agent such as a virus or bacteria.
microbe - microorganisms not visible to naked eye.
placebo - an inactive "fake" substance used in place of medicine or vaccine.
vaccine - a substance containing whole live or killed disease-causing
    microbes. It can be injected or taken orally (by the mouth).
virus - a protein which invades living cells and uses their materials to
    reproduce itself.

Index

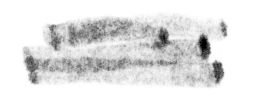

85510